Alkaline Diet Cook Recipes

Delicious Alkaline Plant-Based Recipes for Health & Massive Weight Loss

By Marta Tuchowska

Copyright ©Marta Tuchowska 2015, 2016

www.HolisticWellnessProject.com

www.amazon.com/author/mtuchowska

IMPORTANT

The book is not intended to provide medical advice or to take the place of medical advice and treatment from your personal physician. Readers are advised to consult their own doctors or other qualified health professionals regarding the treatment of medical conditions. The author shall not be held liable or responsible for any misunderstanding or misuse of the information contained in this book. The information is not intended to diagnose, treat or cure any disease.

It is important to remember that the author of this book is not a doctor/ medical professional. Only opinions based upon her own personal experiences or research are cited. THE AUTHOR DOES NOT OFFER MEDICAL ADVICE or prescribe any treatments. For any health or medical issues – you should be talking to your doctor first.

Irresistible Alkaline Dinner Recipes

The Alkaline Diet Lifestyle Cookbook Vol.3

Introduction

Welcome to the third part of *The Alkaline Diet Lifestyle Cookbook* where it's all about healthy and nutritious alkaline diet dinner recipes that are easy to prepare and will give you the energy you deserve. They will also help you understand the basics of the alkaline diet and lifestyle - even if you have never heard about Alkalinity before. It's focused on keeping things as simple and practical as possible.

If you have read *Alkaline Diet Cookbook Vol.1,* or Vol.2 you may want to skip the introduction and go straight to the recipe sections.

This book is for you if:

-you feel like you want to have more energy for life

-you want to learn healthy cooking but don't know where to start

-you are vegan/vegetarian and want to "alkalyze" your way of eating

-you are looking for a natural way to lose weight while giving your body the nutrition it needs

-you want to reduce/eliminate the intake of animal products but don't know how to create recipes that you actually enjoy

-you want to transition towards a natural, wholesome, plant-based, anti-inflammatory diet

-you don't want to spend hours in the kitchen yet want to be able to conjure up healthy and delicious meals that support your health and wellness goals

The Alkaline Diet- The Common Sense Approach

The alkaline diet is a lifestyle that encourages you to give your body the nourishment it needs so that it can work for you at its optimal levels without feeling too exhausted or too acidic. Too much acidity in the body is leading to depression, sickness, and obesity.

Dr. Robert O' Young, Director of Research at the pH Miracle Living Center, says that your fat may be protecting your very life against the acidity in your body. He goes on to make this bold statement.

"There is only one disease: The Constant Acidification of the Body."

What this means is that every disease, including excess weight, is because of a body that is too acidic. These things can make your body too acidic: processed foods, sugar, foods containing gluten and yeast, meat and animal products, stress, alcohol, tobacco, drugs, caffeine, and pollution.

Luckily, the alkaline diet gives us natural tools to fix the problem. I am not talking about overpriced superfoods from overseas that are difficult to find and to pronounce. The simplest methods are always the best and you will be surprised by how healthy you will feel by adding more everyday healing, alkaline foods into your diet (even if you don't follow a strict alkaline diet).

If you attend the root cause of the problem, by implementing a lifestyle rich in alkaline forming foods, it will naturally take care of what plagues you.

My editor, Claire, is a 41-year-old professional woman and a single mom of 3 who suffered from obesity for many years. She just did not have the time to commit to a complicated weight loss program. She made many poor food choices because she was always pressed for time. As a result of her overly acidic body, she experienced tremendous pain from gastric reflux, so much so that her doctor wanted to operate on her.

But once she started following an alkaline plant-based diet (clean, moderate alkaline diet, nothing too strict), she stopped having gastric reflux pain. She began losing weight, and all without feeling deprived and without overdoing or overthinking it. She found she had more energy to get more done each day.

Here are a few simple guidelines that will help you transition towards a healthy, alkaline lifestyle. These are compatible with different nutritional lifestyles (Gluten Free, Vegetarian, Vegan) and it's totally up to you what you choose to focus on:

1) **Eliminate processed foods from your diet and say "no" to colas and sodas** - there are so many additives and preservatives in these foods. They have been known to create hormone imbalances, make you tired, and add to acidity in your body. It's just not natural for humans to consume those conveniently processed foods. The label may even say "low in calories or low in fat"- it will not help you in your long term weight loss or health efforts. In order to start losing weight naturally, your body needs foods that are jam-packed with nutrients. Real foods. Living foods. This, in turn, will help your body maintain its optimal blood pH (7.35) almost effortlessly.

2) **Add more raw foods into your diet**- especially lots of vegetables and leafy greens as well as fruits that are naturally low in sugar (for example, limes, lemons, grapefruits, avocados, tomatoes, and pomegranates are alkaline forming fruits).

3) **Reduce/eliminate animal products** – these are extremely acid-forming. The good news is that there are many plant-based options out there and tons of way to create delicious alkaline-friendly plant-based meals you will love! If I could do it, you can do it too.

4) **Drink plenty of clean, filtered water**, preferably alkaline water or fruit-infused water.

5) **Add more vegetable juices into your diet-** these are a great way to give your body more nutrients and alkalinity that will result in more energy, less inflammation and, if desired- natural weight loss. Vegetable juices are the best shots of health! I have written a book called "Alkaline Juicing" if want to give it a try and want to juice the right way.

6) **Reduce/eliminate processed grains, "crappy carbs" as well as yeast** (very acid-forming). Personally, I recommend quinoa instead (it's naturally gluten-free), amaranth (very nutritious), brown rice, or soba noodles (it's made from buckwheat and naturally gluten-free). You can also use gluten-free wraps or make your own bread. Fruit is also a great natural source of carbohydrates, and great for energy. Plus, they always make a great snack!

7) **Reduce/eliminate caffeine-** trust me - it will only make you feel sick and tired in the long run, and can even lead to adrenal exhaustion (not the best condition to end up in - I have been there). It may seem a bit drastic at first, and yes, I know what you're thinking- there are so many articles out there praising benefits of caffeine and coffee. Yes, I am sure there are, as many people build their business around coffee. This is why there must be something out there that promotes it. At the same time, I agree that everything is good for you in moderation. As long as you have a healthy foundation, you can have coffee as a treat (I do drink coffee occasionally). There is no reason to be too strict on yourself. But...don't rely on caffeine as your main source of energy. Green tea may be helpful too as a transition, but green tea is not caffeine-free either so

don't overdo it. On the other side of spectrum - green tea is rich in antioxidants and a great part of a balanced diet, so it's not that you have to get paranoid about all kinds of caffeine. <u>Moderation is the key</u>. Try to observe your body. Personally, I have noticed that quitting my coffee habits (I used to have 2-3 coffees a day) and replacing coffee with natural herbal teas and infusions have really made my energy levels skyrocket. Now I sleep better, and I get up feeling nice and fresh. I don't need caffeine to keep me awake. I no longer suffer from tension headaches and I feel calmer. Yes, I do have a cup of coffee as a treat sometimes, usually when I meet with a friend, but I no longer depend on it. I choose it; it doesn't choose me. Think about this and how you can apply this simple tip to your life to achieve total wellbeing. Coffee and caffeine in general is extremely acid-forming.

I recently started using an Ayurvedic herb called Ashwagandha. It is known as an adaptogenic herb and it can help you restore your energy levels naturally. I highly recommend you give it a try!

8) Replace cow's milk with almond milk, coconut milk or any other vegan friendly milk (for example quinoa milk, chia seed milk, oats milk-whatever works for you and your stomach) that works well for you. Cow's milk is extremely acid forming and personally, I don't think it makes sense for humans to drink milk that is naturally designed for fattening baby calves not humans. Actually, quitting dairy was one of the best things I have done for myself. I have noticed that even very little milk would cause digestive problems and it was really easy to fix-I quit drinking milk. I also learned about cruelty in the dairy industry which obviously contributed to my decision. The best thing about the alkaline plant-based diet is that you can still have ice cream and other treats- you just make them with no milk/animal products. It's so much healthier and tastier, totally guilt-free. With this approach, there is no need to go hungry or deprived. You focus on abundance of foods and meals that are good for you, delicious and such a choice is also better for the animals and the planet. This is what I call- holistic motivation.

9) **Don't fear good fats- coconut oil, olive oil, avocado oil** etc. are good for you and should replace processed margarines, and artery-clogging trans-fats. This is not to say that you can "drink" them freely. Balance is the key.

Also...

Use stevia instead of processed sugar (stevia is sweet but sugar-free) and Himalayan salt instead of regular salt (Himalayan salt contain some amounts of calcium, iron, potassium and magnesium plus it also contains lower amounts of sodium than regular salt.)

Add more spices and herbs into your diet- not only do they make your dishes taste amazing but they also have anti-inflammatory properties and help you detoxify (cilantro, turmeric, and cinnamon are miraculous).

As you can see, the alkaline diet is a pretty common sense clean diet. Nothing is exaggerated. Nothing is too strict. Nothing is too faddish. Eat more living foods and avoid processed foods. Try to eat more plant based foods. Don't reject it before you have tried it.

Add regular relaxation techniques to the alkaline diet (including yoga, meditation), time spent in nature, adequate sleep and physical activity (we need to sweat out those toxins) and you have a prescription for health. It's strange to me that there are so many people putting the alkaline diet down, however, the general guidelines I have mentioned above are common sense for a healthy lifestyle and I am sure your doctor would agree with it (more natural foods, less processed crap, more relaxation, less stress). This is the gist of the alkaline diet lifestyle. This is what will make you feel nice and rejuvenated and achieve your ideal weight. The problem is that some people are not willing to take those small common sense steps and are looking for a "secret formula" something that will magically help them with no effort at all. I am not judging- I have been guilty of it as well. We all have!

The truth is that whatever changes you want to make in your life (this rule applies not only to health) can be hard as leaving one's comfort zone is difficult, but with time and practise it becomes easy and automatic. Holistic success is about applying what we already know and using the information to better our lives. This is what I call "the secret formula." Information in action.

I always say that I am very open-minded when it comes to different diets. I never claim that what I do is the only path to wellness and health. I prefer to provide you with information and inspiration so that you can create your own way and choose what works for you. Everyone is different. What I teach is based on the alkaline way of living I learned from Doctor Young. However, my alkaline diet may be a bit different than yours and we can still be doing it the right way.

You need to learn to listen to your body and be good on yourself.

Now, with that being said, simply try to adhere to the following recommendations - they will help you understand the gist of the alkaline diet without overwhelming you with complicated pH discussions.

You can easily get started today- simply by making some minor adjustments to your existing diet. Baby steps. I always try to make things simple and easy to apply. Once you apply it - you will feel the amazing benefits of Alkalinity and from there you will want to carry on.

The alkaline diet is not a diet but a lifestyle really. It encourages you to add more alkalizing foods and drinks into your diet so that your body can heal itself naturally. How?

Alkaline Diet Crash Course- Understand the Basics

The pH of most of our important cellular and other fluids (like blood) is actually designed to be at pH of 7.35 (slightly alkaline).

The body has an intricate system in place to always maintain that healthy, slightly alkaline pH level – no matter what you eat. This is an argument that many alkaline diet skeptics use and I get it. It's 100% true.

This is not the goal of the alkaline diet. We just can't make our blood's pH more alkaline or "higher." Our body tries to work really hard for us to help us maintain our ideal pH (7.35). We can't have a pH of 8 or 9. If we did we would be dead.

The entire focus of the alkaline diet is to give your body the nourishment and healing tools it needs to MAINTAIN that optimal 7.35 pH almost effortlessly.

If we fail to do so, we torture our body with an incredible stress! Yes- when the body has to constantly work overtime to detoxify all the cells and maintain our pH it finally succumbs to disease.

Let me just name a few cases of what can happen if we constantly eat an acid-forming diet (also called SAD - Standard American Diet) that is not supporting our body at all. Our body ends up sick and tired of working overtime and may manifest one or more of the following conditions:

-constant inflammation

-immune and hormone imbalance

-lack of energy, mental fog

-yeast and candida overgrowth

 -digestive damage

-weakened bones (our body is forced to pull minerals like magnesium and calcium from our bones in order to maintain alkaline balance it needs for constant healing processes).

In summary, eating more alkaline foods helps support our body so that it can work for us at optimal levels while eating more acidic food doesn't help at all. The alkaline diet is not about magically raising our pH but helping our body rebalance itself by supporting its natural healing functions.

However, it's not only about what we eat - it's also about how we live and what we think. It's not just a diet; it's a lifestyle. If you want vibrant health and alkaline wellness, try to be outdoors more, meditate, laugh, spend time with family and friends, do things you enjoy so that you can de-stress, practise mindfulness...It's not only about nutrition.

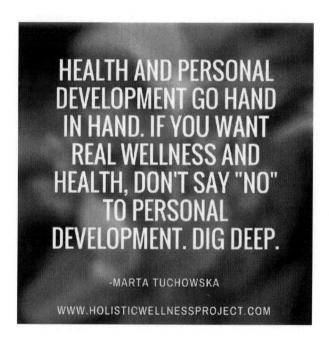

HEALTH AND PERSONAL DEVELOPMENT GO HAND IN HAND. IF YOU WANT REAL WELLNESS AND HEALTH, DON'T SAY "NO" TO PERSONAL DEVELOPMENT. DIG DEEP.

-MARTA TUCHOWSKA

WWW.HOLISTICWELLNESSPROJECT.COM

Over the years, I have also learned that obsessing too much about food or health can be bad. You see - when you are too strict on yourself, this attitude takes away your emotional wellness. Balance is the key: we don't want to be too strict and too obsessed, but we don't want to end up being too lenient as well. You need to be honest with yourself and ask yourself what you can do better and reclaim responsibility for your health and wellness. It's always great to look for that next level, however it's also good to cultivate the sense of gratitude and accomplishment for what we have already managed to change in our diets and lifestyles. Keep learning new recipes and gaining more information about alkaline/vegan/plant based lifestyles. Just keep moving forward, you will get there. Trying is winning!

Oftentimes, it's not about eating less - but about eating right.

Your Free Gifts + Free Alkaline Newsletter

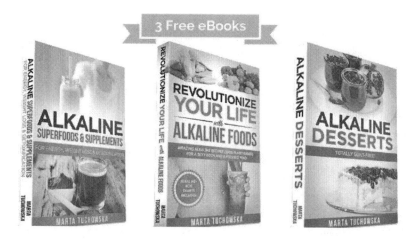

Never heard of the Alkaline Diet and don't know where to start?

I remember when I first learned about the alkaline diet. I was more than confused and sceptical. I wanted to take action but didn't know how. I would spend endless hours online looking for alkaline-acid charts only to find there was way too much contradictory information out there.

I don't want you to feel confused. I also really appreciate the fact you took an interest in my work. This is why I would love to offer you 3 free alkaline diet & lifestyle eBooks + **easy alkaline-acid charts** (printable so that you can keep them on your fridge or in your wallet). They will provide a solid foundation to kick-start your alkaline diet success. You will get all the facts explained in plain English, practical alkaline tips, and yummy, vegan-friendly recipes full of taste, motivational advice, as well as printable charts for quick reference.

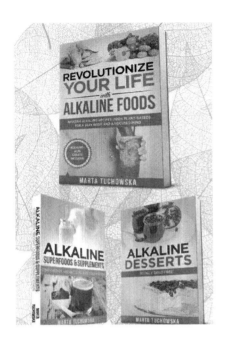

Visit the links below and grab your free eBooks.

Download link:

www.holisticwellnessproject.com/alkaline

The benefits of eating more alkaline & plant-based foods

Since animal products are acid-forming, the alkaline diet is pretty vegan and plant-based in its design. I always try to encourage people to try to stick with vegan options as much as possible- it's fun, it's creative and much more sustainable and better for our environment. Veganism and alkalinity very often overlap and many "alkalarians" are vegans or vegetarians, but we need to remember that vegans stick to their choices not only for their own health, but they also act against animal cruelty and climate changes. People go vegan for a variety of reasons including both their own health, environment, love for animals, even spiritual reasons etc. I believe that an alkaline diet can be a great stepping stone towards veganism.

This is what it did for me; first I reduced animal products, then I decided to go vegetarian (no meat) and finally, a few months ago, I decided to go fully vegan (no animal products whatsoever) and I am loving this lifestyle. I wish I had started it earlier (I lacked information and did not have the right mindset). When I first began my alkaline journey, my own health was my main motivation. I suffered from a really rare eye disease triggered by inflammation and auto-immune system disorders and going alkaline has helped me with my treatment. This is how I became really passionate about it. I finally reached the "almost vegan" stage of my diet and in March 2016, after researching tons of information on veganism, educating myself and learning all the cruelty in the meat and dairy industry, I made a decision to go fully vegan.

As you can see, in my case it was a process. I don't mean to be judgmental, do "holier than thou" or tell people that my way is better than theirs, but since I am experiencing all the fantastic benefits of this alkaline-vegan lifestyle, I want to share this information with as many people as I can.

To sum up - if you can't imagine yourself going vegan at this point, that's fine. Simply try to enrich your diet with more alkaline, plant-based options reducing animal products at the same time. This book will give you dozens of ideas to make a transition a really enjoyable experience. It's not very hard and you will feel healthier and energized as you eat more alkaline and less acid-forming. With the recipes you are just about to discover, I can guarantee that you won't feel deprived or bored. Having plenty of proven recipes is the key to success and the more you learn, the more motivated you will feel.

We also need to keep in mind that the alkaline diet is not about eating 100% alkaline or fully raw. It's not about surviving on cucumbers and kale. Simply try to make about 70% of your diet rich in alkaline-forming foods, it's as simple as that. Whenever in doubt, please check the charts that come as an additional, free resource with this book. You can download and print them at:

www.holisticwellnessproject.com/alkaline

You may want to keep them at hand while shopping, or even going through my recipes.

About the recipes:

- Most ingredients are really easy, everyday and "common sense" ingredients that are easy to find at your local grocery store or supermarket. Occasionally, I may give you some recommendations for natural food supplements or some unusual super foods, but these are not the only path to wellness. The reason why I mention them is for informative purposes, in case you wish to add some new stuff into your diet or you simply like experimenting. Many of those "rare superfood" ingredients can be ordered on-line from Amazon.
- You don't need to be a good cook or a qualified chef to learn those simple and delicious recipes. Honestly, I have never been "spend all her free time in her kitchen" girl (of course there is nothing wrong with that if you are absolutely passionate about cooking, but most people are too tired or too pressed for time). While I do enjoy cooking, as I am attracted to the *creative* part of it as well as health benefits that I can rip off if I cook the right way, I always try to make the whole process as simple as possible. I am a big fan of automation as well and so I like batch-cooking to make sure I always have some healthy options to fall, back on. Let's be real - everyone can have a bad day and cooking may seem like a mission. This is why having something that is already waiting for you that you prepared in advance is a great

life saver. This is especially true if you are on a busy schedule or have a big family to feed.

- You don't need any fancy kitchen equipment to get started on my recipes. While having a good blender or food processor helps and so does food spiralizer, you can also use a simple hand blender and a knife. Add to it chopping boards, oven, pans and pots and you have all you need.
- Most of my recipes are quick to prepare- give it 20 minutes or less and you have a delicious and nutritious meal that supports your health and fitness goals.

Again, let's remember that the alkaline diet is not about eating 100% alkaline. Let's aim for 70%. It's so much easier, right? The remaining 30% can be acidic foods, but this not justify processed foods that need to be buried forever. Your number one goal should be to eliminate all processed convenience foods. Then keep trying different foods and recipes and observe what works for you.

I always say that you need to listen to your body. On top of that, any drastic changes in your diet should be discussed with your doctor.

The Alkaline Diet Made Easy. Even for Busy People

As soon as you try my recipes and eat more alkaline, you will soon start noticing all the benefits of eating a diet jam-packed with vitamins, minerals, natural protein, fibre, healthy fats as well as free of artificial sugar, gluten and other processed foods.

Now, here's why many people fail with the alkaline diet and healthy eating in general. I am not judging as I have been guilty of it many times. It stems from the fact that a person gets passionate about health, but tries to do it all at once or doesn't know where to start. You need a good strategy to fall back on.

It's simple, if you only rely on willpower your goals probably are:

-just ignore all the cravings and hold on

-eat only healthy alkaline foods and be strong and stick to it- if I have to survive on salads so be it!

Unfortunately, this strategy is not a plan I recommend. It may not last for too long unless you are a super strong-willed person.

Here's the problem with this approach and I have faced it so many times:

You end up eating the same stuff all the time, and you get obsessed about foods. So you stress too much about the whole healthy eating thing. It means that you are constantly wondering what you're going to eat or what you just ate. Anxiety and guilt trips form part of this self-torture and it seems like health and wellness success is farther and farther away.

Then you think about your family and friends. They think you're a rabbit! They eat some yummy stuff and you are right in front of them with another boring salad (let me guess-iceberg lettuce, tomatoes and cucumber?).

It's not hard to fail in this scenario. In fact it's pretty normal. It would be weird if you didn't fail while following this crazy strategy. The risks could be that you don't get proper nutrition you need (you just worry too much about your pH) and your emotional wellness just leaves you.

The good news is that Marta is here to show you how to do it right with her recipes so that you eat a clean, balanced plant-based diet inspired by the alkaline diet and compatible with your current nutritional lifestyle. You enjoy it and so it's not that hard for you to create a healthy lifestyle. Moreover, it's cool to get new skills in the kitchen and treat your family and friends to healthy and delicious meals.

Alkaline Diet- Common Questions

Are lemons acidic or alkaline?

This is my favourite question and if you are a beginner, it's normal you are asking it. The answer is very simple: it's all about the effect that the food has on our body after it has been consumed, not before. <u>It doesn't matter to us what pH they have in their natural state (before they have been eaten).</u> Lemons are full of alkaline minerals and at the same time they don't contain sugar which makes them one of the very few alkaline fruits.

Remember to get your starter's guide and food list at:

www.holisticwellnessproject.com/alkaline

They will save you confusion.

What about Protein?

The choice to avoid/reduce the consumption of meat and other animal-derived products is becoming increasingly accepted among the general public. Restaurants and supermarkets are catering for vegans and those opting for an alkaline diet ever more than in the past offering a wide selection of delicious and vegan-friendly products. Some of these foods have been crafted to imitate certain things that you may wish to continue to enjoy, just in a novel, plant-based form, instead. Such things include non-dairy ice cream and yogurt, for example. Other foods, of course, are naturally vegan-friendly with even their conventional forms being entirely of plant origin.

Although the issue of finding vegan-friendly, alkaline products and restaurant items is becoming less of a problem in big cities and healthy food stores, this does not mean that this availability translates into a simple and easy life of making everyday vegan dishes at home. It's this particular challenge that we are now going to tackle with the help of the book you now hold in your hands. Making tasty and nutritious alkaline friendly dishes at home doesn't need to be difficult or expensive, and you'll soon be able to use the recipes in this book to prove it to yourself once and for all.

Plant-based protein:

- Hemp (You can use hemp powder in your smoothies.)
- Green leafy veggies (One cup of cooked spinach has about 7 grams of protein. Kale is pretty much the same.)
- Quinoa (It has about 9 grams of protein per cup.)

- Almond Butter (It is great with gluten-free breads and wraps. Two tablespoons of almond butter is about 8 grams of protein.)
- Other choices include: lentils (great in salads), beans and chickpeas
- Nuts and seeds (for example sunflower seeds)

HEALTH BENEFITS OF VEGAN/ALKALINE/PLANT-BASED DIETS:

- lower cholesterol levels

-lower blood pressure,

-lower rates of Type 2 diabetes,

-lower risk of death from heart disease,

-lower overall cancer rates

-less acidity in the body

-natural weight loss

-clean skin

-healthier immune system

-improved digestion

Recommended resources:

www.nutritionfacts.org by Doctor Michael Greger.

His website offers tons of great information as well as scientifically proven approach to plant based diets.

Do I have to give up my favourite foods forever?

Luckily, you don't. The mere thought of having to give everything up is just unbearable, right? Don't try to be perfect. Focus on progress. For example, in my opinion, people do much better if they try to be 70-80% great and 20-30% relaxed than if they try to be 100% perfect- all the time. This rule also applies to other goals, not only health. This approach is so much easier when you are just starting out!

It is also important to remember that you can still have your favorite foods (ice cream, pizzas, even burgers) in their vegan, alkaline versions! This is great news! Again, it's not that you have to survive on green smoothies alone.

Besides, if you try to be perfect (for example, you try to stick 100% to smoothies and salads) you may experience many negative emotions (deprivation) that are not healthy. In fact, stressing too much about food or life in general, can be very acid-forming.

Now it's not a secret that raw foods are more alkaline than cooked foods. But you can still be alkaline even if you don't follow a 100% raw food diet (you can if you want to, but it's not the only path to wellness and health). Personally, my number one rule is to keep it all plant based, and 70-80%

alkaline. I also like combining cooked foods with raw foods. My body tells me what's good for me and my digestion.

You don't have to give up your life. You can still go out with friends and socialize. You can still have that glass of wine or an occasional coffee.

Alcohol is highly acid-forming, but you can enjoy a couple of drinks on social occasions every now and then. I am not talking about getting drunk of course, but there is nothing wrong with having an occasional drink with a friend and having a laugh. The problem is when you feel you need a drink because you can't deal with stress or you need it to boost your confidence (I have been there, I am not judging). In that case, I recommend you resort to meditation, hypnosis, NLP, yoga, natural remedies, and guided meditation. You can also check out my blog that is full of holistic wellness and relaxation tips:

www.HolisticWellnessProject.com

There are many options out there that can help you create a new, stronger, more stress-free and more confident version of yourself with long-term success.

So back to acid-forming foods and drinks, just remember-moderation is the key. It's not that you will have to give up all the acidic foods forever. At the same time, I am not saying you should be indulging in unhealthy foods all the time. Just follow your own pace.

However, I strongly recommend you give up sodas and other artificial drinks as well as chemically processed foods, and convenience foods. They do not bring you closer to your goals at all. There are healthier snacks out there, you can make your own fries and crisps, and you can experiment with fruit infused water that is a great alternative to sodas and also much, much cheaper.

Also don't try to do it all at once. Set simple goals. For example: this week I will replace sodas with fruit infused water. Action plan: get the recipes and ingredients. Done? Great. Next step. Repeat the process, for example: this week I will try to drink one alkaline smoothie a day and have some salad with my lunch/dinner. Done? Great. Create the next step. For example: this week, I will get committed to physical activity or yoga. Only one step at the time. Baby steps. Here and now. I call it- mindful motivation.

Now, with all of that information out of the way, it's time to start looking at some delicious recipes. Each category includes a number of tasty dishes with a little description telling you what's so good about it from a nutritional/lifestyle point of view. You'll also find easy to follow instructions for each dish, so you'll never have a moment's hesitation when making beautiful and healthy dishes for you and your loved ones.

Shall you happen to have any questions or doubts about this book (or you want to say hi) just email me at:

info@holisticwellnessproject.com

I love hearing from my readers!

Important:

I am not a doctor/therapist or a scientist, and I am not giving you any specific advice related to serious health problems. So if you happen to have any specific health questions, remember to talk to your doctor or health professional first. Please read a full disclaimer at the beginning of this book.

As a wellness coach I help people with **motivation**, habits and **practical holistic self-care tips** so that they can create a healthy lifestyle with long-term benefits that allows them to prevent numerous illnesses and lose weight in a healthy way. I call it a holistic lifestyle design, something that I am absolutely passionate about and honestly, I am even more passionate about helping you being passionate about it as well. This is my mission and this is what I stand for. I want to help you work on your body, mind and soul so that you can create success in all areas of life. It all starts with energy and vibrant health.

Also, remember that you can also use my recipes as templates to create your own. If there is any ingredient you don't like or your body can't tolerate - skip it. We need to listen to our body and be selective if necessary. Everyone is different and so are their nutritional preferences. Follow your way (but try to keep it plant based as much as you can, sorry I had to make this remark).

Read on and enjoy!

Don't forget to download your free complimentary eBooks at:

www.holisticwellnessproject.com/alkaline

Recipe Measurements

I love keeping ingredient measurements as simple as possible-this is why I stick to tablespoons, teaspoons and cups.

The cup measurement I use is the American cup measurement. I also use it for dry ingredients. If you are new to it, let me help you:

If you don't have American Cup measures, just use a metric or imperial liquid measuring jug and fill your jug with your ingredient to the corresponding level. Here's how to go about it:

1 American Cup= 250ml= 8 fl.oz

For example:

If a recipe calls for 1 cup of almonds, simply place your almonds into your measuring jug until it reaches the 250 ml/8oz mark.

I know that different countries use different measurements and I wanted to make things simple for you.

Translations (US-UK English)

Eggplant=Aubergine

Zucchini=Courgette

Cilantro=Coriander

Garbanzo Beans=Chickpeas

Navy Beans-=Haricot Beans

Aragula=Rocket

Broth=Stock

Amazing Alkaline-Friendly Dinners

Eating alkaline is easier than you can imagine, especially if you have a set of delicious and easy-to-make recipes. Evening is a time of the day when we are very prone to all kinds of unhealthy temptations, simply because we feel a bit tired and very often stressed. Luckily, the alkaline diet can take care of you with a whole variety of tasty and nutritious dinner recipes.

With this recipe book, you will be looking forward to celebrating dinner time with your family, friends and, of course, your favorite healthy foods. My number 1 suggestion is: always try to have some healthy, guilt-free snacks for late afternoon and early evening. It can be a real lifesaver and can actually make you reconsider the desire to order some pizza or take away food. Since most people are busy or tired in the evenings, it's better (and safer) to make sure that you cook in batches (for example on weekends), plan your meals and always have some veggies that are ready to grab (washed and chopped). This is a fantastic plan to minimize the time you spend in the kitchen or shopping. Planning is the key.

Many of my readers and clients told me that evening time was the most difficult time to "stay healthy" as they all had uncontrollable food cravings and just felt like giving in to eating bad. This is something I can definitely relate to as I had this problem in the past and it would spoil all my alkaline diet efforts. The solution is quite simple:

1. Stop "going hungry". You see, many people focus on eliminating certain foods first instead of adding. The way I see it is like this: focus on adding more alkaline foods first and then start gradually eliminating acidic foods that do not support your health goals.
2. Do not skip breakfast and always eat lunch.
3. Be sure to carry some alkaline snacks, like nuts and seeds, with you.
4. Try to have a small mid-afternoon meal. Here in Spain, where I currently live, they call it "merienda," in Poland, where I am originally from, they call it "podwieczorek" (such a difficult word, I know!). I usually grab a smoothie, a simple veggie wrap or some homemade gluten-free bakes. I usually have 5 meals a day (yes!), breakfast, mid-morning snack, lunch, mid-afternoon snack and dinner. Golden rule - it's not about eating less; it's about eating right. If you follow this rule, you will make it to evening time feeling nicely energized and really motivated to carry on a healthy track. Heck, with this 5 meals a day routine, I can even have a nice evening walk before or after my dinner. The energy you get from eating more alkaline is amazing, and I am absolutely passionate about helping you experience it in a doable, easy, fun and practical way!

Once you've learned some of the recipes in this section, dinner will never be a bore again. In many parts of the world, animal products are hard to come by and people have had to rely on naturally vegan foods by necessity rather than choice. We can make the most of these recipes and their invariably nutritious content by using them to make tasty evening meals for everyone in the family.

Alkaline Dinners

Vegetable Paella

Unlike most forms of paella, this dish is completely vegan-friendly. It contains everything you could ask for from a single dish and can be eaten with great pleasure at any time of year.

Serves: 4-6

Ingredients:

- 3 tbsp. olive oil
- 1 onion, finely chopped
- 1 eggplant, finely chopped
- 1 zucchini, finely chopped
- 1 red bell pepper, finely chopped
- 3 cloves of garlic, finely chopped
- 2 tomatoes, chopped
- 1 tsp smoked paprika
- 1 1/3 cups paella (Arborio) rice
- 6 cups boiling water
- Pinch of saffron
- 2/3 cup green beans, finely chopped
- 2/3 cup peas

Instructions:

1. Add the olive oil to a large frying pan and sauté the onion, eggplant, zucchini and red bell pepper over a medium heat until golden.
2. Add the garlic and cook for 1 minute, until fragrant.
3. Add the tomatoes, rice and smoked paprika.

4. Stir and then add half the water along with the saffron and some salt and black pepper to taste.
5. Stir the mixture and then cover and increase the heat.
6. Cook at a high heat for 10 minutes, ensuring that you don't burn anything.
7. Add the remainder of the water, stir and cover. Reduce the heat to medium and cook for 20 minutes. Do not stir at this point.
8. Add the green beans and peas for the final 5 minutes of cooking.
9. The rice ought to be *al dente* (=firm) when ready. Leave to stand for 5 minutes and then serve while still hot.
10. Enjoy!

Tofu in Black Bean Sauce

While many of you may choose not to consume soya products, it can be an important protein source for those who do enjoy the occasional piece of tofu. As such, this recipe has been included in this book with the intention of inclusivity in mind. The wide variety of mushrooms used in such dishes (even though not alkaline) can be a great source of vitamin D.

Serves: 4
Ingredients:
- 1 cup dried mushrooms (shiitake mushrooms are particularly delicious)
- 3/4 cup boiling water
- 1 cup fresh firm tofu
- 3 tbsps. coconut oil
- 4 green bell peppers, chopped
- 1 large fresh chili pepper, deseeded and sliced
- 2 cloves of garlic, sliced
- 1 tbsp. cornstarch

+Boiled brown rice or quinoa to serve on the side

For the sauce:
- 2 tsp black bean sauce
- 3 tbsps. Bragg Liquid Aminos
- 1 tbsp. hoisin sauce
- 1 tbsp. tomato purée

Instructions:
1. Place the mushrooms in a bowl and add the boiling water. Leave them for 30 minutes to become reconstituted.

2. Reserve the water from the mushrooms. Slice the mushrooms and add the sauce ingredients.
3. Drain the tofu and wrap in paper towels to absorb any excess liquid. When you are ready, cut them into 3/4 inch pieces.
4. Add the sunflower oil to a wok placed over a high heat. Add the mushrooms, green bell pepper, chili and garlic and stir fry for 2 minutes. Be sure not to burn the garlic.
5. Add the sauce mixture and stir the contents of the wok continuously for about 2 minutes, until the sauce is thickened.
6. Add the cornstarch to the cool mushroom water, stir, and then pour into the wok.
7. Stir the mixture over the wok until thick, and then add the tofu, stirring until it has been coated with the sauce and warmed through.
8. Serve immediately with a side of boiled rice.

One Pot Beans

Beans are one of the most important sources of protein for those of us following a vegan way of life, and this dish makes them simply delicious. This recipe is great for when those cold, winter nights are drawing in.

Serves: 4
Ingredients:
- 2 tbsps. olive oil
- 2 vegetable stock cubes, crumbled
- 2 onions, chopped
- 2 apples, peeled and grated
- 2 carrots, grated
- 3 tbsps. tomato purée
- 1 cup water
- 1 tsp dried oregano
- 1 tsp ground cumin
- 2 cups red kidney beans, pre-cooked
- Salt and black pepper to taste

Instructions:
1. Preheat the oven to 350°F. (175 Celsius)
2. Sauté the onion, stock cubes, apple and carrot in a frying pan over a medium heat for 5 minutes, stirring constantly.
3. Mix the tomato purée into the water. Add this, the dried oregano, and ground cumin to the sautéed mixture and stir well.
4. Cover and simmer for about 2 minutes.
5. Add the red kidney beans, stir, and pour the whole mixture into a casserole dish.

6. Cover and cook in the oven for about 40 minutes. Add a little extra water if the mixture starts to look dry.
7. Serve while still hot.

Sweet Potato Cottage Pie

Cottage pie is one of those homely classics, perfect at any time of year as a bit of comfort food. This version consists of an all vegan filling and uses sweet potato as the topping, rather than the more conventional white potato. This way, you get a source of starchy goodness with a healthy dose of vitamin A to top it off. That's not something the average white potato could do!

Serves: 6
Ingredients:
For the filling:
- 1 tbsp. olive oil
- 1 leek, finely chopped
- 1 parsnip, diced
- 1 carrot, diced
- 1 celery stalk, diced
- 2 cloves of garlic, minced
- 2 cups canned tomatoes
- 1 tbsp. tomato purée
- 2 cups green lentils, cooked, drained and rinsed
- 1 cup frozen peas
- Salt and black pepper

For the topping:
- 4 medium sweet potatoes, chopped
- 1 tsp vegan margarine or coconut oil
- ¼ cup fresh dill, chopped

Instructions:
1. Sauté the onion, leek, carrot and parsnip in olive oil until the vegetables begin to soften.

2. Add the garlic to the frying pan and season with salt and black pepper to taste.
3. Add the tomatoes, tomato purée and simmer for 20 minutes. Add some water if the consistency is too thick.
4. To make the sweet potato mash, boil the sweet potato in salted water for 20 minutes, until it is soft. Drain and mash with the vegan margarine.
5. Stir the dill into the mashed sweet potato and return to the heat, cooking gently for around 5 minutes, until the mixture begins to firm up. Set aside when ready.
6. Preheat the oven to 360°F. (180 Celsius).
7. Add the drained and rinsed green lentils to the tomato sauce. Add the frozen peas and cook for 5 minutes until fully heated through.
8. Transfer the filling to an 8 inch baking dish. Top the filling with the sweet potato mixture, ensuring that it is covered completely.
9. Bake for around 30 minutes, until the cottage pie is bubbling in the oven.
10. Leave the dish to cool for around 10 minutes, then serve and enjoy.

Sweet Potato Wedges with a Twist

Very easy dish that helps you sneak in some green, alkalizing and hydrating veggies in the form of spiralized zucchinis.

Servings: 4 to 6
Ingredients:
- 6 large sweet potatoes, peeled and cut in wedges
- 4 tablespoons coconut oil
- 1 teaspoon smoked paprika + other spices of your choice (curry also works great!)
- Himalayan salt to taste
- 2 zucchinis, sliced very thinly with a spiralizer

Instructions:
1. Preheat the oven to a temperature of 450°F (230 Celsius) and line two rimmed baking sheets with parchment.
2. Mix the sweet potatoes with some coconut oil adding the spices and Himalayan salt.
3. Place the potatoes in a single layer on top of the rimmed baking sheets.
4. Start baking and keep stirring occasionally. When almost done (after about 15 minutes) add the spiraled or sliced zucchinis and keep baking for 5 minutes more until soft.
5. Cool for 5 minutes and serve with some greens on side.

Easy Vegan Burger

This is my favorite vegan-alkaline fast food!

Servings: 4
Ingredients:
- 2 large red bell peppers, chopped
- Coconut oil
- Salt and pepper to taste
- 4 vegan sandwich buns, preferable gluten-free or sprouted, toasted
- 4 tablespoons fresh basil pesto
- 1 cup fresh arugula

Instructions:
1. Stir fry the red bell peppers in coconut oil adding Himalayan salt and spices of your choice.
2. Set aside when ready.
3. Spread some pesto on the top half of each sandwich bun.
4. Place the stir-fried red bell peppers onto the bottom half of each sandwich bun.
5. Top with fresh arugula and the top half of the buns.
6. Serve warm.
7. Enjoy!

Easy Red Pepper Hummus

This hummus can be a real life-saver. If you are too busy to cook or too tired after work, you can just satisfy your hunger in a healthy way. Hummus is great to serve with raw veggies as well as in all kinds of wraps.

Servings: 10 to 12
Ingredients:
- 1 cup chickpeas, cooked, rinsed and drained
- 1/4 cup of roasted red peppers, chopped
- 3 cloves minced garlic
- ½ jalapeno, seeded and minced
- Himalayan Salt and pepper to taste
- 4 tablespoons olive oil
- Water, as needed
- 2 tbsps. fresh cilantro
- Juice of 1 lime

Instructions:
1. Combine the chickpeas, cilantro, roasted red pepper, garlic and jalapeno in a food processor and blend until super smooth.
2. Add in some olive oil, lime juice, and water to achieve the desired consistency and blend again.
3. Add Himalayan salt and pepper to taste, mix well and serve as a dip with some raw veggies or sprouted bread/wraps. Enjoy!

Alkaline Comfort Tomato Soup

Tomatoes are miraculous and highly alkalizing. They are one of my favorite alkaline common-sense super foods!

Serves: 2-4
Ingredients:
- 3 cups of fresh tomatoes, peeled (immerse in some warm water to get the peel off)
- 4 leeks thinly sliced
- 6 garlic cloves, minced
- 2 tablespoons coconut oil
- 1 cup vegetable broth
- 1 can coconut milk or almond milk
- Salt and fresh pepper or other spices to taste

Instructions:
1. Using a large saucepan, sauté leeks in some oil (medium heat) until translucent.
2. Add garlic and stir together for 1 minute. Switch off the heat.
3. In the meantime, blend the peeled tomatoes in a blender.
4. Add the mixture to your saucepan and put on low heat. Stir well.
5. Add coconut milk, vegetable broth, salt and spices.
6. Simmer on low heat until warm and serve.
7. Enjoy!

Easy Tomato Salad

The easiest way to get more alkaline is to simply add more raw foods into your diet, especially alkaline fruits and vegetables. It's not that you have to survive on salads alone, but if you just choose to serve some salads with your main meals, you will certainly see a difference.

Serves: 4
Ingredients:
- 1 small shallot, thinly sliced
- 4-5 medium tomatoes, sliced
- 2 cucumbers, peeled and spiralizer
- ½ cup alfalfa sprouts
- 6 medium basil leaves
- Himalayan salt
- Freshly ground pepper
- Juice of 1 lime
- Olive oil or avocado oil

Instructions:
1. Combine all the ingredients in a salad bowl, toss well and enjoy!
2. If you want, you can add some protein.
3. Enjoy!

Alkaline Ginger Soup

Nutrition and simplicity very often go hand in hand. This soup is great not only as an easy dinner recipe, but also as a side dish or nourishing, alkaline tonic.

Serves: 4
Ingredients:
- 10 carrots, peeled and chopped
- 1 onion, diced
- 4 tablespoons minced ginger
- 3 cups vegetable broth
- 2 tablespoons coconut oil
- Himalayan salt and black pepper to taste

Instructions:
1. Heat up some coconut oil in a large pan (medium heat) and fry until translucent.
2. Reduce the heat to low heat, add carrots and ginger. Keep stirring.
3. Now add vegetable broth, and simmer until carrots are tender.
4. When done, place through a blender.
5. You can serve it with some protein of your choice.
6. It's great in winter, but you can also serve it cold, as a summer refreshment.

Alkaline Mineral Broth

Another amazing mix of common-sense superfoods in a common-sense recipe. There is no need to splurge on exotic superfoods that are very often hard to pronounce and to find. I recently recommended this recipe in one of my newsletters, and the feedback I got was amazing. If you want to receive more recipes from me (as soon as they are created or as soon as I discover them), remember to join our alkaline wellness club (free newsletter) at:

www.holisticwellnessproject.com/alkaline

Serves: 6
Ingredients:
- 4 medium sweet potatoes
- 1 cup zucchini, chopped
- 1 cup cabbage, chopped
- 1 cup celery, chopped
- 5 carrots, chopped
- 1 cup collard greens, chopped
- 1 cup kale, chopped
- ½ cup onion, minced
- 1/2 cup parsley
- ½ cup beets
- 5 cloves garlic
- ½ cup flax seeds
- A few inches of ginger root
- Himalayan salt, olive oil and black pepper to taste
- 3 liters of water
- Optional: Any other veggies you have around the house.

Instructions:
1. Place the veggies in a big pot and add water.
2. Bring to boil using low heat and simmer 4 hours or more.
3. Add Himalayan salt, olive oil and spices.
4. Strain and keep the broth.
5. Drink at least 1 cup per day.
6. Variations: If you like thicker soups instead of broths, you can blend everything together in a blender.
7. In case you decide to strain it, you can keep the veggies for curry stir-fries and vegetable pancakes.

Alkaline Thai Style Potatoes

Great recipe for those who love Asian flavors!

Serves: 3
Ingredients:
- 3 medium sized sweet potatoes or yams
- ½ cup coconut milk
- ¼ cup smooth almond butter (raw, unsweetened)
- 1 tablespoon wheat free tamari sauce
- 1 tablespoon chili sauce
- 1 teaspoon olive oil
- ½ teaspoon red pepper flakes
- 2 minced garlic cloves
- 2-3 drops liquid stevia
- Pinch of Himalayan salt
- 2 tablespoons coconut oil
- 1 cup chickpeas, cooked and drained
- 1 red bell pepper, chopped
- ¼ teaspoon garlic powder
- Salt and pepper, to taste
- 2 green onions, finely chopped

Garnish:
- 1 tbsp. cilantro, finely chopped
- ¼ chopped cashews

Instructions:
1. Preheat oven to 400 degrees Fahrenheit (200 Celsius).
2. Make several holes with a knife or fork in each sweet potato. Bake in the oven for an hour or an hour and fifteen minutes, wrapped tightly in foil.

3. In the meantime, blend together garlic clove, red pepper, olive oil, garlic sauce, tamari sauce, coconut milk and almond butter using a food processor or a blender. Add 2-3 drops of stevia to sweeten.
4. Pour some coconut oil into a sauté pan using medium heat and add red pepper, onions, chickpeas as well as salt and pepper. Sauté for 5 minutes.
5. Turn off the heat when soft.
6. Fill each half of a sweet potato with mixture, garnish with cilantro and cashews.
7. Enjoy!

Alkaline Couscous

This is a very simple solution for busy people and the dinner leftovers can make a great take-away lunch for the next day!

Serves: 2
Ingredients:
- 1 cup couscous (preferably gluten-free)
- 1 yellow onion, peeled
- 1 cucumber
- 4 tomatoes
- 1/2 red chili
- ¼ cup fresh mint leaves
- ¼ cup fresh coriander leaves
- 1/4 cup fresh parsley leaves
- 1 /2 cup pureed tomato
- 2 tablespoons olive oil
- 1 small lemon, juice and zest
- 1 teaspoon ground cumin
- 1 teaspoon paprika
- Himalayan salt to taste
- powdered black pepper
- boiling water

Instructions:
1. Place couscous in a big bowl.
2. Add enough boiling water to cover the couscous. Be careful not to add too much water.
3. Stir in some salt and spices. Cover and set aside.
4. In the meantime, chop the veggies (onion, tomatoes, and chili) and herbs (parsley, coriander and mint).
5. Now take a couscous bowl and stir in the tomato puree until well coated.

6. Add all the veggies, herbs and spices mixing well.
7. Sprinkle over some olive oil, lemon zest and juice, and add salt and pepper.

Easy Root Salad

This is yet another delicious, easy to make, vegan friendly option that is fantastic for detoxification. It can make a simple dish if you are not too hungry, or serve as a side dish.

Serves: 2
Ingredients:
- 4 fresh beetroots, peeled and sliced thinly
- 3 carrots, peeled and spiraled
- 1 heart celery, with leaves, sliced
- ½ cup arugula
- ½ cup radishes, diced
- 1 fennel bulb, (save the roots for later use)
- Olive oil and lemon juice or alkaline chili dressing (see recipe below)
- Himalayan salt and black pepper

Instructions:
1. Place beets, celery heart and leaves, radishes, arugula and fennel in a salad bowl.
2. Toss well and sprinkle over some lemon juice and olive oil (or alkaline chili dressing from the next recipe).
3. Season with Himalayan salt and pepper. Enjoy!

Alkaline Chili Dressing

This simple recipe is a great way to spice up all your salads, dips, sauces and even wraps.

Ingredients:
- 2 red chilies (fresh, not dried)
- 1/2 cup extra virgin olive oil
- 3 tablespoons lemon juice
- 1 tablespoon lime juice
- 1/4 cup fresh mint leaves, leaves picked and finely chopped
- A few tablespoons coconut milk
- Himalayan salt
- Black pepper

Instructions:
1. Peel the chilies; take out and discard the seeds.
2. Finely chop the chilies and combine with lemon juice, coconut milk, mint and olive oil.
3. Add salt and pepper to taste.
4. Sprinkle a bit to your regular salad dressing. Careful, it's hot!

Easy Sweet Potato Curry

This recipe is a real pleasure for your taste buds!

Serves: 2

Ingredients:

- 1 cup chickpeas, cooked and drained
- 2 tbsp. olive or coconut oil
- 4 medium sized sweet potatoes, peeled and cubed
- 1 onion, diced
- 1 tbsp. ginger powder
- 1 tbsp. curry powder
- ½ cup vegetable stock
- 1 can full fat coconut milk
- salt and pepper to taste

To garnish:

A handful of cilantro and mint leaves

To serve:

Arugula, spinach or other greens to serve on side.

Instructions:

1. Add 1 tbsp. olive or coconut oil to a skillet and heat up on medium-high heat.
2. Add the onions and cook until translucent.
3. Reduce to low/medium heat and add ginger, garlic and curry powder, and pinch of Himalayan salt cooking for another 2 minutes.
4. Now add the potatoes and vegetable stock. Keep stirring.
5. When almost soft, add chickpeas and coconut milk. Stir again. Turn off the heat when potatoes are done.
6. Garnish with cilantro and mint leaves and serve with some greens on side. Enjoy!

Alkaline Tacos

This vegan friendly recipe combines the amazing benefits of black beans (high in fiber and vegan protein) and broccoli (great for liver detoxification, just like all green foods). While very few people are naturally attracted to broccoli, this recipe makes it more appealing.

Serves: 2-4
Ingredients:

Broccoli:
- 1 large head of broccoli, sliced into small florets
- 3 tbsp. olive oil
- salt and pepper to taste

Black Beans:
- 1 tbsp. olive oil
- 1 white onion, finely chopped
- 2 garlic cloves, minced
- 2 tbsp. organic tomato sauce
- ¾ cup black beans, cooked and rinsed
- 2 cups vegetable broth (you can use alkaline mineral broth from previous recipes)
- 1 tsp. ground cumin
- ½ tsp. chili powder

Tacos:
- 8 gluten-free tortillas

Taco Sauce:
- 1/3 cup vegan mayonnaise (check out the bonus recipes at the end of this book)

- 2 tbsp. lemon juice
- 3 tbsp. hot sauce of your choice
- salt and pepper to taste

Instructions:

1. Preheat oven to 400 degrees Fahrenheit (about 200 Celsius).
2. Massage broccoli with some coconut oil.
3. Add salt and pepper to taste, and place broccoli on a big baking dish.
4. Roast until golden brown (about 30 minutes). Remove once half way through to turn.
5. In the meantime, take a sauté pan, heat some coconut oil over medium heat and add onion and garlic.
6. Season with a pinch of salt, and cook for a few minutes until soft.
7. Add tomato paste, cumin and chili powder. Stir well.
8. Now add black beans and veggie broth.
9. Simmer for 10 minutes so that the beans take the flavor.
10. In the meantime, whisk all the sauce ingredients together and set aside.
11. Once everything is done, prepare for serving. Top each tortilla with black bean mixture and broccoli. Sprinkle over some sauce and enjoy!

Easy Cucumber Bean Salad

Great salad recipe for hot summers, or as a side dish throughout the year.

Serves: 2

Ingredients:

- 2 medium large cucumbers, peeled and sliced (or spiraled)
- 2 carrots
- 2 big ripe tomatoes
- 1 red or green bell pepper, finely chopped
- 1 cup red onions, diced
- ½ cup cilantro, finely chopped
- ½ cup cashews
- ½ cup garbanzo beans, cooked and drained
- ½ tsp. Himalayan salt
- ½ tsp. garlic powder
- ½ tsp. chili powder
- ¼ tsp. ginger powder
- ¼ tsp. cumin
- 1/8 tsp. turmeric
- Cilantro leaves to garnish
- Juice of 1 small lime

Instructions:

1. Mix all the salad ingredients in a big salad bowl.
2. Toss well adding spices, salt and olive oil.
3. Sprinkle over some lime juice. Garnish with fresh cilantro leaves.
4. Serve and enjoy!

White Bean Avocado Sandwich

This recipe is a great "vegan fast-food" option with an alkaline twist. It also works well for lunch. It's not that you have to quit bread forever. Just choose healthy bread options (for example gluten-free, multi-grain) and of course, don't overdo it.

Serves: 2
Ingredients:
- ½ cup white beans, mashed
- 2 tbsp. olive oil
- Pinch of Himalayan salt and black pepper
- 4 slices of multi-grain or gluten free bread (wraps also work great)
- A few onion rings
- 1 carrot, peeled and thinly sliced
- 1 avocado, peeled, pitted and thinly sliced
- 2 handfuls of sprouts (alfalfa or soy sprouts - you decide)

Instructions:
1. Lay your bread slices or wraps of choice open, and add some bean mixture.
2. Top with onion rings, carrots, sprouts and avocado.
3. Close your sandwiches, serve and enjoy!

Easy Quinoa Bowl

This recipe combines the alkalizing benefits of avocado (excellent source of healthy fats) and kale (which is high in Vitamins K, A and C.)

Serves: 4
- 1 cup quinoa, cooked
- 1 bunch kale stems removed and finely chopped
- ½ cup lemon juice
- 2 tbsp. olive oil
- ½ jalapeno pepper, diced
- ½ tsp. cumin
- salt to taste

Avocado salsa:
- 1 avocado, sliced
- 2 tomato, chopped
- 1 jalapeno pepper, diced
- ½ cup cilantro leaves, chopped
- ¼-1/2 red onion, finely chopped
- 1 lemon, juiced

Instructions:
1. Prepare your dressing by whisking together lemon juice, olive oil, jalapeno, cumin and salt.
2. Place kale leaves in a salad bowl and massage it well with your salad dressing.
3. In a separate bowl, mix together all avocado salsa ingredients and set aside.
4. In serving bowls, distribute equal amounts of quinoa and kale.
5. Top with avocado salsa. Enjoy!

Alkaline Spinach Soup

Great for a well-deserved liver detox!

Serves: 4-5
Ingredients:
- 2 tbsp. coconut oil
- 2 leeks, white parts, chopped
- 4 garlic cloves, peeled and minced
- 4 celery stalks, chopped
- 3 medium heads of broccoli, chopped
- 8 cups of veggie broth
- 3 cups spinach leaves, chopped
- 1 cup parsley, chopped
- salt and pepper to taste

Instructions:
1. Heat some coconut oil in a pot over medium heat.
2. Add garlic and leeks, and fry until just slightly browned.
3. Add broccoli and celery, stirring for a few minutes.
4. Now add vegetable stock and bring everything to a boil on low heat.
5. Remove from heat when broccoli gets tender.
6. Then, add the spinach and parsley, just to heat it slightly.
7. Place the mixture through a food processor and blend until smooth.
8. Season to taste, serve and enjoy. Personally, I love it creamy, with some coconut oil.

Amazing Raw Tomato Soup

This recipe is super easy and you can also enjoy it between your meals for more alkaline energy!

Serves: 4-6
Ingredients
- 6 big tomatoes, peeled
- 2 carrots
- 1 inch fresh ginger, peeled
- 3 garlic cloves, minced
- 2 tablespoons olive oil
- 1/2 cup vegetable broth
- ½ cup coconut milk (full fat)
- Salt and fresh pepper to taste

Instructions:
1. Blend all the ingredients in a food processor or a blender.
2. Serve raw or slightly warmed.
3. Personally, I like to throw in some stir-fried veggies, chickpeas or quinoa.
4. This recipe is highly alkalizing and so if you decide to eat something that is not alkaline, it's always good to have it as a side dish to achieve alkaline balance.

Raw Spinach Salad

Spinach is miraculous and if you are serious about going alkaline, you should consider eating more of it. This recipe helps you do it in an easy and enjoyable way.

Serves: 4-6
Ingredients:
- ¼ cup strawberries, halved
- 8 cups spinach leaves, washed and chopped thinly
- 4 tbsp. almonds, crushed
- ½ onion, finely chopped
- 1 grapefruit, peeled and chopped (sprinkle over some stevia if you find it hard to eat grapefruit)
- 1 avocado, peeled, pitted and chopped
- 2 tablespoons chia seeds for more nutrition
- Olive oil and Himalayan salt to taste

Instructions:
1. In a salad bowl, combine all the salad ingredients and stir well.
2. Sprinkle over some olive oil and Himalayan salt.
3. Enjoy!

Alkaline Thai Kale Salad

This simple recipe is an easy and delicious way to sneak more kale into your diet.

Serves: 4

Ingredients:

- 3 cups kale leaves, stemmed
- 1 large sized red onion, thinly sliced
- 2 tablespoons coconut aminos
- Juice of 2 limes
- ½ cup coconut milk
- 2 jalapeño peepers, diced
- Zest of 1 lime
- 2 orange sweet peppers, diced
- 3 cloves garlic, peeled, minced
- Coconut oil

Instructions:

1. Sauté the red onion slices in some coconut oil.
2. Add the garlic clove, sweet peppers and jalapeño slices to the onions.
3. Stir fry until slightly golden.
4. Blanch the kale leaves in a pot of boiling water. Drain and set aside.
5. In the meantime, mix the coconut aminos, lime zest and lime juice with the coconut milk. Set aside.
6. Mix kale leaves and the veggies. Drizzle the coconut milk dressing on top to serve.
7. Enjoy!

Apple and Celery Root Salad

Apples in salads are great and make it much tastier!

Serves: 2-4

Ingredients:

- 1 medium red apple, peeled and diced
- 2 tablespoons of *vegan or* home-made mayonnaise (recipe in the bonus section)
- 1 medium sized celery root, peeled and grated
- 4 tablespoons of chopped almonds
- Juice of 1 lemon
- 2 carrots, sliced
- 2 cucumbers, sliced
- 2 tablespoons of coconut cream
- 1/4th cup of minced fresh parsley leaves
- Olive oil and lime juice
- Himalayan salt and pepper to taste

Instructions:

1. Combine all the salad ingredients in a salad bowl.
2. Toss well. Stir in some mayonnaise and give it a thorough mix again.
3. Sprinkle over some olive oil and lime juice.
4. Season with Himalayan salt and black pepper to taste.
5. Enjoy!

Artichoke Salad

Artichokes are miraculous and really good for your liver. They also make delicious salads!

Serves: 2

Ingredients:

- 2-3 brine dipped artichoke hearts, halved
- 2 cups of fresh arugula leaves
- ½ cup of almond powder mixed with cashew powder
- 1 red onion, sliced
- Half cup soy sprouts

Dressing:

- A few tablespoons homemade mayonnaise check the recipe in the bonus section)
- 2 tablespoons olive oil
- Juice of half a lemon

Instructions:

1. Combine all the salad ingredients in a salad bowl.
2. Toss well. Stir in some mayonnaise and give it a thorough mix again.
3. Sprinkle over some olive oil and lime juice.
4. Season with Himalayan salt and black pepper to taste.
5. Enjoy!

Summer Veggies Salad

Servings: 2
Ingredients:

- 1 red organic beetroot, peeled and sliced
- 6 radishes, sliced
- 1 orange
- 1/2 of a red onion, peeled and sliced
- Zucchini, sliced or spiraled stir-fried in coconut oil
- optional: 1 small sized kohlrabi, sliced
- 1 red pepper, deseeded and sliced
- ¼ cup of almonds

Dressing:

- 2-3 tablespoons olive oil
- 2 teaspoons of fresh oregano, chopped
- 1 clove of garlic, peeled and finely chopped
- 2 drops liquid stevia
- 2 tablespoons coconut milk
- 1 tablespoon of fresh parsley leaves, chopped
- Fresh juice of 1 lemon
- Pinch of Himalayan salt

Instructions:

1. Combine all the dressing ingredients, stir well and set aside.
2. Combine all the salad ingredients in a salad bowl.
3. Toss well and sprinkle generously with the salad dressing.
4. Enjoy!

Green Papaya Salad

Papaya is great for digestion and has a plethora of anti-inflammatory benefits. I remember visiting the Canary Islands and indulging in papaya smoothies and salads there because papaya was really cheap and easy to get. I wish I was there now. Holidays are always too short, right?

Serves: 2

Ingredients:

- Cup of mixed fresh lettuce leaves of your choice
- Green papaya, julienned
- ¼ cup radish slices
- A few tablespoons of raw cashew nuts
- ½ cup cherry tomatoes

Spicy Dressing:

- 1 tablespoon maple syrup
- 2 tablespoons of coconut milk or almond milk
- 1 red long chili, seeded and finely chopped
- Juice of 2 limes
- 1 small clove of garlic, peeled and minced

Instructions:

1. Mix all the dressing ingredients in a small bowl and set aside.
2. In the meantime, combine all the salad ingredients in a larger salad bowl.
3. Toss well. Stir in some spicy dressing depending on your taste preferences and give it a thorough mix again.
4. Sprinkle over some olive oil and lime juice.
5. Season with Himalayan salt and black pepper to taste.
6. Enjoy!

Grapefruit Avocado Salad

Both grapefruits and avocados are considered super alkaline foods. Imagine the combined energy powers...

Serves: 4

Ingredients:

- 2 whole avocados, peeled, pitted and sliced
- 2 tablespoons of extra virgin olive oil
- A pinch of Himalayan salt
- ¼ cup almond powder or crashed almonds
- 2 grapefruits, peeled and sliced
- A few raisins (optional)

Instructions:

1. Combine all the salad ingredients in a salad bowl.
2. Toss well. Sprinkle over some olive oil.
3. Season with Himalayan salt.
4. Enjoy! This salad is extremely alkaline and will help you balance your ph level.

Easy Pomegranate Salad

Pomegranates are highly alkalizing fruits and taste great in salads.

Serves: 2
Ingredients:
- 1/2 cup of fresh rocket leaves
- Juice of 1/2 fresh lemon
- 2 oranges, peeled and halved horizontally
- A few tablespoons cashew powder
- 1 whole pomegranate, seeded
- A few small sprigs of mint, leaves separated
- Some olive oil

Instructions:
1. Combine all the salad ingredients in a salad bowl.
2. Toss well.
3. Sprinkle over some olive oil and lemon juice.
4. Enjoy!

Easy Yummy Spinach Salad

Quick and easy detox recipe with amazing anti-inflammatory nutrients from fruit, veggies, and protein.

Serves: 2
Ingredients:
- 2 cups spinach leaves, chopped
- 1 avocado, peeled, pitted and sliced
- 1 peach, pitted and chopped
- 1 cup tomatoes, sliced
- ½ cup almonds
- 2-4 slices smoked tofu, chopped
- 2 tablespoon olive oil
- Juice of ½ lemon
- Himalayan salt and black pepper

Instructions:
1. Mix everything well in a large bowl.
2. Sprinkle over some olive oil and lemon juice.
3. Season with Himalayan salt and black pepper.

Alkaline Pizza

Who said you can never have pizza again? It's all about creating a healthy, clean, alkaline versions of your favorite meals. Enjoy! This is a really amazing comforting meal that makes sure you get enough veggies into your diet!

Ingredients:
For the Alkaline Crust:
- 1.5 cup spelt or almond flour (spelt is not gluten free, if you want to keep it gluten free, use almond or white rice flour instead).
- 1/2 teaspoon of Himalayan salt
- 1 tablespoon baking powder
- 1/2 cup alkaline water
- 2 tablespoons olive oil (extra virgin)

Alkaline Tomato Pizza Sauce:
- 4 medium tomatoes
- 2 garlic cloves
- ½ teaspoon Himalayan salt
- 1 tablespoon Italian seasoning (oregano and basil)
- 1/8 cup olive oil

Toppings:
1.5 cup of veggie mix (I like all kinds of peppers mixed together)

- Fresh kale (optional), raw or stir-fried

- A few onion rings

You can also add other veggies of your choice

Instructions:
-First, preheat your oven at 375 degrees Fahrenheit (190 Celsius).
1. Start with a crust: in a bowl, mix all the dry ingredients in a bowl.
2. Add the wet ingredients and mix well.
3. Now knead the dough with your hands. It should be sticky. Keep working on it for about 5 minutes adding more flour if necessary.
4. Cover it with a damp piece of paper towel and set aside.
5. In the meantime, get the sauce ready: simple blend all the sauce ingredients in a blender.
6. Optional: you may want to stir-fry the veggies before using them for topping.
7. Now, it's finally time to roll out the dough onto a pan and spread the sauce to make sure the dough is equally covered.
8. Add the toppings (the veggies you have chosen)
9. Now, it's time to wait for it impatiently; bake for about 20 minutes (at the above mentioned 375 degrees Fahrenheit). Enjoy!

Cucumber Salad (Alkaline-Paleo)

A very simple way to conjure up a quick dinner salad!

Serves: 4
Ingredients:
- 2 cups cooked quinoa
- 3 cucumbers, peeled and sliced
- 1/2 red onion, thinly sliced
- 3 tbsp. lime juice
- 2 tablespoons olive oil
- 3 tbsp. coconut yoghurt or coconut cream (thick coconut milk is also fine)
- Himalayan salt and pepper to taste
- 2 avocados, peeled, pitted and sliced
- ½ cup blueberries
- 1 tsp. chopped cilantro

Instructions:
1. Whisk or thoroughly stir together all ingredients in a bowl.
2. Sprinkle over some lime juice, coconut yoghurt and olive oil.
3. Mix well, season with salt and pepper and enjoy!

Alkaline Pesto Pasta with Veggies

Zucchini noodles are just fantastic and a great option on gluten-free, grain-free diets. This recipe is light and refreshing, perfect for hot summer evenings. Really alkalizing. You can never go wrong with this one.

Serves: 4
Ingredients:
Pesto:

- 2 cups fresh basil
- ¼ cup freshly grated vegan parmesan cheese (optional)
- ½ cup olive oil
- juice of half a lemon
- 1/3 cup pine or walnuts
- 3 garlic cloves
- salt and pepper to taste

Veggie Pasta

- 2 cups zucchini, spiraled into noodles
- Coconut oil

Instructions:

1. First, prepare pesto sauce. Begin by toasting pine or walnuts, heat a bit of olive oil in a pan on medium heat, add nuts, and stir constantly until browned. Remove from heat.
2. Add all pesto ingredients to a food processor and blend until smooth. Season to taste as needed. Set aside.
3. Heat up some coconut oil in a medium-size skillet and add spiraled zucchini. Stir-fry on low/medium heat for about 5 minutes until soft.
4. Pour over the pesto sauce and stir well. Serve and enjoy!

Bonus Recipes

Homemade Mayo

Vegan Option:

Mix: half cup almond or coconut milk, 2
tablespoons fresh lemon juice, 1 tablespoon Dijon
mustard, half cup of olive oil, pinch of salt and pepper.
You can experiment with the consistency by adding
some almond powder and coconut oil. Enjoy!

Alkaline Yummy Coconut Macaroons

These are dangerously addictive and really healthy. Perfect for evening time when you have an after-dinner "sweet tooth." Coconut is an alkaline fruit and spices like cinnamon and vanilla not only add to your wellbeing but also have anti-inflammatory and soothing properties. You don't need to feel guilty about this one.

Ingredients:

- 1 cup coconut butter (may be hard to find, but not impossible, I get my from health store or from Amazon.com)
- 1 cups shredded, unsweetened coconut
- A few drops if liquid stevia
- 1 tsp. vanilla
- dash of cinnamon and nutmeg

Instructions:

1. Preheat oven to 325 degrees Fahrenheit (160 Celsius), and line a baking sheet with parchment paper.
2. Heat the coconut butter (low heat and small pot) stirring energetically so that it's completely melted.
3. Mix all ingredients together in a bowl, until well combined.
4. Dough should be thick, you can always add a bit more shredded coconut to make it thicker.
5. Form small cookies and place them on the baking sheet.
6. Bake for about 15 minutes (keep checking as these are easy to burn so don't leave them unattended).
7. Allow your macaroons to cool for 20 minutes, serve and enjoy.

Chia Flax Dessert

This is a great, guilt-free dessert option for you to enjoy. Everyone loves chocolate and this recipe is a healthy, dairy-free and gluten-free alternative that is totally compatible with the alkaline diet.

Serves: 1-2

Ingredients:

- 1 cup berries (organic if possible)
- 1 ½ cup coconut milk
- 1 tbsp. chia seeds, ground
- 1 tbsp. flax seeds, ground
- 1 tsp. unsweetened cocoa powder
- 2 drops liquid stevia
- 1 tsp. cinnamon

Instructions:

1. Blend using a blender and enjoy!
2. Serve immediately or chill in a fridge.

Conclusion

Thank you for reading!

I hope that with so many alkaline-friendly recipes you will be motivated and inspired to start your journey towards vibrant health and total wellbeing.

Remember, the beauty of incorporating alkaline foods into your daily diet is that you are making simple, yet sustainable changes that will work for your wellness long-term.

In reducing processed foods from your diet, you are working to prevent many potential diseases such as cancer, diabetes, arthritis and many more. On top of that, you are providing your family with important nutritional foundation that they need to create a life full of happiness, energy and fulfillment.

If you enjoyed my book, it would be greatly appreciated if you left a review so others can receive the same benefits you have. Your review can help other people take this important step to take care of their health and inspire them to start a new chapter in their lives.

At the same time, you can help me serve you and all my other readers even more.

I'd be thrilled to hear from you. I would love to know your top 3 recipes.

BIG THANKS!

Your 3 FREE eBooks + Alkaline Wellness Newsletter

Don't forget to download your free eBooks.

They are waiting for you at:

www.holisticwellnessproject.com/alkaline

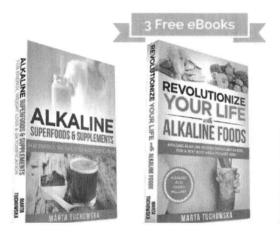
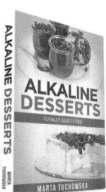

Let Me Help You

If you have any questions, doubts, or you find my instructions confusing and need more guidance, please e-mail me. I am here to help. Don't be shy. I am also looking for feedback. If you have any suggestions that can help me improve my work, please let me know and I will take an immediate action to serve you better in the next editions.

info@holisticwellnessproject.com

More Alkaline & Wellness Books by Marta:

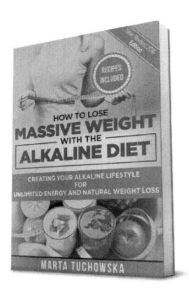

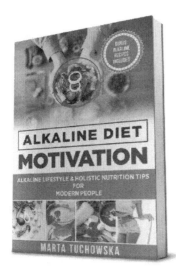

You will find them + many more at:

www.holisticwellnessproject.com/books/

FINALLY- LET'S KEEP IN TOUCH:

www.instagram.com/Marta_Wellness

www.facebook.com/HolisticWellnessProject

www.twitter.com/Marta_Wellness

www.pinterest.com/martaWellness/

I wish you wellness, health, and success in whatever it is that you want to accomplish.

With lots of LOVE and positive energy,

Marta Tuchowska

Printed in Poland
by Amazon Fulfillment
Poland Sp. z o.o., Wrocław